HEALTHCARE
COST ACCOUNTING
Practice And Applications

JEFFREY A. GOTTLIEB

ISBN 0-930228-67-7

Table of Contents

Chapter One

Why Cost Accounting?

Are the following scenarios familiar?

The director of marketing comes into your office and describes an opportunity to bid on a contract that will increase volume. She asks how large a discount can be offered in order to bid competitively for the referrals. If the hospital's bid is not competitive, it could lose several hundreds of thousands of dollars of income opportunity.

Your hospital has 60 signed PPO/HMO contracts; five represent 80 percent of the total PPO/HMO revenue. The board of directors wants a report immediately from the hospital president detailing profitability by contract.

A new program is being evaluated. Gross and net revenues are reasonably estimated based upon volume and payer-type distributions. However, the services provided cover the broad spectrum of nursing and ancillary departments. How much confidence can be put in the cost estimates when comprehensive final product cost accounting has not been completed? Medicare's cost-to-charges ratios could be used, but how valid are the ratios out of the context of the rules and regulations of the Medicare program?

One of the hospital's largest volume admitters of Medicare patients is also contributing more to the contractual expense than is any other physician. The hospital is considering motivating the physician to move his patients elsewhere. Before proceeding, are you sure of the positive or negative impact of the contribution margin on the bottom line?

The finance and marketing departments are analyzing the effect of establishing centers of excellence so as to significantly change the mix and volume of services and patients. Do you have the best information to determine the potential profits or losses from such a service restructuring?

The chief executive officer has been asked to present to the next board of directors' meeting the net gain to the hospital of subsidizing graduating residents' private offices within the local community. Is the information available to determine the profit contribution from expected admissions from specific physician specialties?

Budgeting time has arrived. Would it not be ideal to develop a prospective budget model based upon payer-type and case-mix assumptions instead of just patient day projections?

The hospital board has requested a financial review of the utilization review function. Is the information available to reasonably assess the cost savings?

A manager reports this year that his department is much more efficient than it was the prior year. Is standard cost variance analysis to be performed at the unit level to confirm this perceived performance improvement?

These scenarios illustrate common business and planning opportunities for using cost accounting. These opportunities can be summarized in the following categories:

Strategic Planning (Strength, Weakness, Opportunity and Threat Identification)

Effective PPO/HMO Contracting

Program Expansion/Divestiture Analysis

Resource Utilization/Productivity Monitoring and Management

Flexible Budgeting

Capital Planning Analysis

Executives and middle management in health care are under tremendous pressure to increase profitability through improved financial controls, marketing, planning and increased operational efficiency. These pressures are primarily being applied by government and other payers in the form of DRGs, HMOs, PPOs, IPAs and a veritable alphabet soup of contractual arrangements. The two unified goals of these changes are to introduce competition into the healthcare industry and to reduce the payment per purchased unit of service. If hospitals are to prosper in the new environment, many changes must occur.

One critical change is to develop timely and accurate information for decision making. Such information requires quality supporting data. The resulting information must be meaningful, relevant and able to reduce uncertainty.

The most meaningful information within our industry answers the question: "What is the cost of producing distinct healthcare services?" This information becomes highly relevant when used for decision making—as for a new program.

The hospital industry is one of the few major industries that does not know how much it costs to produce its products. While charge and cost reimbursement did not encourage the examination of unit costs for specific services, with the rapid movement toward prospectively determined payment mechanisms, this concept of cost awareness becomes critical to the survival of hospitals.

Although it is popular to compare our industry unfavorably with manufacturing when decrying the lack of healthcare cost information, we should be aware that cost accounting in the manufacturing environment is also experiencing change. The manufacturers' impetus for change is also competition: the influx of quality lower-priced imports.

Now that manufacturers want to reduce the level of inventory on hand and be able to compete on price as well as quality, discrete product cost information—such as variable and fixed cost—becomes highly relevant and as important as traditional inventory-valuation costing systems. Thus the manufacturers are in a similar position as healthcare providers: they need more information but existing systems do not accommodate this need.

The major objective of this primer is to motivate the healthcare provider to make that modest but intelligent leap forward into developing the basic cost information required for effective management decisions.

To achieve that objective, this primer describes the issues and processes involved in developing a cost accounting data base and in implementing systems for translating the raw data into useful information. Although the material is based upon actual experiences, there are no absolute rules for success. The reader is advised to modify appropriately the basic guidelines to his or her organization's unique characteristics and cost accounting expertise. This primer is not intended to be a complete theoretical textbook on cost accounting and standard costing, but rather a blueprint for successfully building a cost accounting system.

Recognizing that the significance of cost accounting lies not in the numbers themselves but in their applications, a significant portion of this primer is dedicated to the benefits and reasonable expectations of cost data in such activities as cost/benefit analysis, budgeting, cost variance analysis, PPO/HMO contract management and case-mix management.

This primer is written with the intent of making cost accounting less confusing and less mysterious by conceptually discussing the processes and the applications. However, sufficient detail is provided so that cost accounting planning can be immediately initiated by the designated finance manager. It is highly recommended that the planning process include a selected review of other cost accounting literature as well as discussions with other providers who have started or completed procedural and final product cost accounting.

Chapter Two
Organizational Requirements and Structure

Regardless of how a hospital approaches cost accounting, both executive and middle management must be committed to the process and goals. That commitment is obtained through educating management, planning, setting clear objectives and achievable timetables, and selecting a qualified implementation team.

Executive Commitment

Because detailed and comprehensive cost accounting is relatively new to the healthcare industry, it is critical to have executive support at the beginning and throughout the process. The two members of executive management whose support is most important are the Chief Executive Officer and the Chief Financial Officer. If the organization includes a Chief Operating Officer, that individual's commitment is also needed.

A high level of commitment is required because information and data will be collected at the department level. Department management cooperation can become uncertain without explicit direction from executive management. Lack of department support can both lengthen the project and result in lower quality data.

Scope of Project

After executive management has fully committed itself to the project, it is necessary to develop a detailed workplan. In defining the scope of the project, the workplan will include:

—Appropriate use of the 80/20 rule
—Desired level of costing detail
—Determination of departmental involvement
—Choice of costing methodologies for each department
—Organizational structure
—Cost accounting system selection criteria and implementation
—Project time schedule and milestones

Implementation Staff

The selection of a quality cost accounting staff or consultants is one of the critical factors of success. Most important, the individual(s) responsible for managing the cost accounting process must be knowledgeable not only about the cost components of your organization's services and procedures but also about the applications of the cost data base itself. This familiarity with the organization's overall cost accounting objectives will contribute toward achieving the desired results.

An "optimal resume" for the person directing and managing the cost accounting function would include:

—Masters in business, healthcare administration or equivalent
—Undergraduate degree in either accounting or industrial engineering or equivalent
—Five-plus years experience in financial management or analysis
—Two-plus years experience in cost accounting
—Three-plus years experience in the healthcare industry
—Certification as either a management accountant or a public accountant

The likelihood of securing such an individual in industry or consulting is minimal, considering that the opportunities for extensive healthcare cost accounting experience have been few.

In lieu of these specific degrees and years of experience, the following skills could be accepted:

—An excellent knowledge of management accounting (for example, cost accounting, budgeting, etc.), financial planning and analysis, and financial accounting (generally accepted accounting principles)
—Knowledge of healthcare organizational structures, financing, and alternative systems of delivery
—Excellent written and verbal communication skills, and the ability to translate complex processes into easily understood steps for implementation

The type of individual described in the above optimal resume is known as a management accountant. Until recently, financial management of the healthcare industry was skewed toward primarily financial reporting and business office management. The financial "insulation" provided by predictable government and private reimbursement, coupled with the lack of competition, resulted in minimal demand for extensive management accounting skills.

The role of the management accountant is internal. A management accountant will participate in such processes as budgeting, cost accounting, pricing decisions, lease vs. buy decisions, capital investment analysis, and so on. The academic degree most likely to provide the theoretical background would be a masters in business administration. The Certificate in Management Accounting exam, as administered by the National Association of Accountants, is generally recognized as a test of an individual's comprehensive understanding of management accounting principles.

The role of the financial accountant, on the other hand, is more external. It is usually defined within the constraints of the requirements of the "public." Although the data requirements for financial accounting and management accounting will overlap, the methods for summarizing that data into information will vary because of the differing requirements of the public and management.

Financial accounting (reporting) must conform to generally accepted accounting principles promulgated by recognized bodies such as the Financial Accounting Standards Board (FASB). The education providing the conceptual understanding of financial accounting is usually an undergraduate college program in accounting. The Certificate in Public Accounting administered by the American Institute of Certified Public Accountants is the highest recognition of an individual's understanding of generally accepted accounting principles in relation to financial accounting.

In the workplace, these roles become blurred by actual responsibilities and tasks as well as individual talent, career goals, and ambition. And though cost accounting is a major foundation of management accounting, the subject will often be more thoroughly covered at the standard cost level by an undergraduate program in accounting than by a masters degree in business. However, the MBA program will often cover the general applications such as budgeting and investment analysis much more thoroughly.

Accordingly, when considering the individuals to be responsible for cost accounting, the organization should be aware of their skill base and experiences, as well as their orientation toward the applications of the developed information. Regardless of academic background, probably one of the most important considerations is healthcare cost accounting experience.

Consultants

Many organizations will consider the use of consultants. While it is advisable to use experienced consultants for planning and guiding the project, there is a definite "brain drain" effect if outside assistance is overused. Those individuals who are involved "hands-on" not only learn a great deal about the cost and operating structure of the hospital, but also greatly appreciate the limitations, benefits and opportunities of the cost accounting data base. There are tremendous recurring benefits, particularly to the CFO, for keeping that knowledge and skill set in-house.

Consulting is no longer subsidized by the Medicare program to the extent it was prior to the implementation of the DRG payment mechanism. Before 1983 it was possible to have as much as 50 percent or more of consulting fees (depending upon the extent of Medicare utilization of services) reimbursed through the Medicare cost report as administrative and general expense.

Yet consulting services will continue to be necessary because they provide specific training and broad experience and because no hospital can hire in-house expertise in every possible management or technical field. However, the changing healthcare market does require that consulting services be used more prudently. A cost accounting endeavor is no exception.

Cost accounting consulting services can cost anywhere from $10,000 to well over $200,000 depending upon hourly fees, acquisition of computer systems, extent of intermediate and final products costed and level of costing accuracy. Considering the need for periodic updating of the cost accounting data base, the ongoing purchase of consulting fees can become quite expensive during these times of fewer resources. Accordingly, an approach should be considered that reaps the full benefits of quality cost accounting while minimizing the expense.

Increasingly, consultants are being used by hospitals as project leaders directing in-house staff. Recognizing that hospital finance/accounting staff have the potential for developing cost accounting data, there should be few economic reasons for using outside consultants on a permanant basis. The following are benefits of a consultant-staff project approach to cost accounting:

—Minimizes consulting fees
—Adds to the skill base of in-house staff
—Permits hospital staff to continue the project in subsequent years with less or no assistance from outside consultants
—Reduces the inefficiency and consequences of trial and error by internal staff
—Allows the organization to receive benefit from the experience and technical skills of the consultant as well as from his leadership in planning, scheduling and coordinating the project.

The process of cost accounting and its applications should benefit the institution, and not become an annuity for the consultant. Hospitals need the existing staff to be able to maintain, improve and convey the required cost accounting information to middle and executive management.

Scheduling

Project milestones will vary from institution to institution and there are no hard rules for their establishment. For instance, a hospital that seeks only to define costs as either fixed or variable for a limited number of departments may complete the project in three to four months or less. A hospital desiring to study all departments and break costs out by direct and indirect fixed and variable components for salaries, supplies and capital related items may take ten to fourteen months to complete the project.

Factors affecting the relative scheduling of each milestone are as follows:

—Depth and experience of the cost accounting staff
—Systems and applications selected
—Desired quality and complexity of the cost accounting data
—Support and cooperation provided by executive and middle management

The schedule of major milestones (Exhibit 1) might be appropriate for a hospital planning to do intermediate and final product costing implemented by a staff of skilled healthcare managers with little or no practical cost accounting experience.

Management Education

Critical to the success of the project are education and commitment. Commitment is obtained from middle management by the visible commitment of senior management and by the discernible competence of the implementation staff. Education serves two purposes. Though the first is to ensure that correct and accurate information is being supplied to the implementation staff by middle management, the education process itself also communicates the implementation staff's skills and knowledge.

A sample agenda for a two-session middle management course is shown as Exhibit 2.

Exhibit 1: Milestone schedule

Activity	Relative Time Frame
1. Cost accounting research (for example, literary search, read articles, textbooks, etc.)	▬
2. Development of cost accounting workpapers, educational materials, etc.	▬
3. Presentation to executive management regarding goals, objectives, schedule approach, management commitment	▪
4. Middle manager orientation (for example, 30-minute overview at regular general management meeting)	▪
5. Middle management educational/ training sessions	▬▬
6. Development of cost standards by implementation staff, in cooperation with middle management	▬▬▬▬▬
7. Review of intermediate product costs for reasonableness	▬▬▬
8. Final development of intermediate product costs	▬▬
9. Use of intermediate product cost data with case-mix and decision support systems	▪

Exhibit 2: Agenda for middle management course

Session One: Theory (1 Hour)

1. Objectives of 1st and 2nd session
2. Objective of product line accounting
3. Cost concepts and examples
   —Fixed cost
   —Variable cost
   —Direct cost
   —Overhead cost
   —Indirect cost
   —Average cost
   —Incremental and marginal cost
4. Questions.

Session Two: Practice (2 Hours)

1. Cost accounting expectations of organization
2. Cost accounting resources and tools available
3. How standard costing differs from historical costing
4. Example: Developing an intermediate and final product cost standard
5. Example: Application of product cost standards
6. Alternate methods for developing product costs
7. Questions.

Organizational Lines of Responsibility and Reporting

Different organizational structures have been suggested for cost accounting. Typically, the function reports directly to the Chief Financial Officer because of the obvious accounting/financial nature of the process. Exhibit 3 shows one of many structural approaches. Obviously, the structure must match the characteristics of each organization.

Exhibit 3: Cost accounting organizational structure

Executive Management Council, (CEO, COO, CFO, VPs)	Determines need for cost accounting. Provides initial policy statements as to objectives and expected outcomes. Mandates middle management commitment to the success of the project.
Chief Financial Officer or Controller	Accountable for project's success and maintenance of data. Selects implementation team/consultants. Plays lead role in determining project's goals and objectives. Manages data base for use by finance, marketing, planning, utilization review, etc.
Cost Accounting Implementation Staff and/or Consultants	Plans and schedules. Educates executive and middle management. Works with middle management in developing intermediate (for example, procedure) product standards. Utilizes cost accounting case-mix software to determine intermediate and final product (for example, DRG) cost. Reports to CFO periodically as to project status.
Department (Middle) Management Nursing Ancillary Support	Works with implementation staff developing intermediate product costs and standards. Updates data on a periodic basis. Uses information for budgeting, department program planning, etc.

Chapter Three
Cost Accounting Concepts

Cost Accounting Defined

Whereas cost accounting covers a wider range of subjects, the cost accounting objectives of most hospitals today are limited to "cost finding." Cost finding, simply described, is:

> The study of cost behavior and
> the identification of total (full) costs
> and those components that comprise total cost.

It should be noted that cost finding is only an initial step. Costing should not be performed solely to identify the cost of services and products, but rather applied to some analytical process so as to achieve a business objective, such as profit maximization.

Many disciplines and processes can benefit from a quality cost accounting data base. This includes budgeting, new program and capital project evaluation, inventory management, pricing, addition or divestiture of a product line, profitability determination by group of purchasers (payers), cost control, and overhead and corporate expense allocation.

Management Accounting Cost Concepts

An understanding of basic management accounting cost concepts is critical to successful cost accounting. This section concisely reviews various cost concepts. The definitions may be as short as a single sentence or as long as several paragraphs. Most of the concepts will be discussed in more detail in subsequent sections. For further explanations the reader is referred to the bibliography.

ALLOCATED INDIRECT COST. Overhead or indirect costs that are allocated to direct patient care departments in order to determine the full cost of providing services. The allocation process requires two inputs: the set of costs to be allocated and the selection of a statistical base on which to allocate those costs.

Example: A hospital has five departments. Three of the departments are revenue-producing and two are overhead. The five departments and their budgeted expenses are illustrated on the next page:

Department	Revenue Producing	Overhead	Budgeted Expenses
Medical Records		X	$ 300,000
Housekeeping		X	400,000
Clinic	X		700,000
Routine Care	X		1,000,000
ICU	X		2,000,000

To allocate Medical Records and Housekeeping expenses, it is necessary to use a reasonable measure of each department's utilization of the overhead services. For this example, chart requests and net square footage have been chosen, respectively, as the statistics for Medical Records and Housekeeping. The following is the allocation process.

Medical records
(Determination of allocated costs by department)

Revenue Producing Department	Number of Charts	Percentage of Total Charts	Costs to be Allocated	Allocated Costs
Clinic	6,000	60%	$300,000	$180,000
Routine Care	3,000	30%	300,000	90,000
ICU	1,000	10%	300,000	30,000
	10,000	100%		$300,000

Housekeeping
(Determination of allocated costs by department)

Revenue Producing Department	Net Square Feet	Percentage of Square Feet	Costs to be Allocated	Allocated Costs
Clinic	10,000	50%	$400,000	$200,000
Routine Care	7,000	35%	400,000	140,000
ICU	3,000	15%	400,000	60,000
	20,000	100%		$400,000

The above percentages are the proportion of total volume used by each patient service department (for example, 6,000 charts divided by 10,000 total charts equals 60 percent). Allocated costs are the proportion of statisticial units multiplied by the total overhead costs to be allocated (for example, 60 percent multiplied by $300,000 equals $180,000).

The total cost of each revenue-producing department is the sum of the direct expenses plus the allocated expenses. For the clinic this would be $700,000 direct expense plus $180,000 for medical records plus $200,000 for housekeeping services for a total full cost of $1,080,000.

ASSIGNABLE COSTS. See DIRECT COST.

AVERAGE COST. Cost divided by volume. Example: From the preceding page, the budgeted direct expense for the clinic is $700,000, while the total cost is $1,080,000. If budgeted units of activity are 10,000 visits, then the average direct expenses are $70 per visit ($700,000 divided by 10,000) and the average total expenses are $108 per visit (1,080,000 divided by 10,000).

BUDGET. A plan of expected results measured in financial terms.

COMMON COSTS. See JOINT COST.

CONTROLLABLE COST. An item of cost can be considered controllable if the amount is significantly influenced by the actions of the service manager. Most variable costs are controllable. When the hospital is viewed as a single entity, all costs must be considered controllable by the hospital chief executive officer.

COST ACCOUNTING. The accumulation of cost and related data to be used for financial reporting and business decision making.

COST CENTER. An organizational unit, recognized in the chart of accounts, for which relevant expenses and revenues are accumulated.

COST-TO-CHARGE RATIO. A ratio of departmental full cost to total charges. Used by the Medicare program for inpatient reimbursement prior to implementation of DRGs. Limited to use for procedural costing because intermediate product pricing may be based on factors other than cost, such as competition.

DIRECT COST. The cost clearly traceable to a unit of activity or cost center, such as direct labor costs or direct material costs.

The time spent by a laboratory technician to perform a unique procedure is the direct labor cost of the procedure. The pathology department manager is a direct cost to the department and an overhead cost to each test. The manager's services are not directly traceable to individual pathology tests as are the technician's time and salary.

Most often procedural direct expenses can be assumed to be variable, but this may not be true, for example, where direct staffing cost is incurred even in such circumstances of excess capacity or no activity.

FINAL PRODUCT. Product or service purchased by consumer, manufacturer, PPO/HMO, etc. Typically an accumulation of intermediate products (for example, lab tests) bundled to produce an end product (for example, DRG).

FIXED BUDGET. See STATIC BUDGET.

FIXED COST. A cost that is independent of the level of activity.

FLEXIBLE BUDGET. A budget projecting expenses at various levels of activity.

FULL COST. The total cost of a department or procedure is the sum of direct and indirect costs.

HISTORICAL COST. Actual costs incurred in prior time periods by department or product for various types of resources, such as labor and materials. Can be used as a tool for projecting future costs.

INCREMENTAL COST. Analogous to marginal cost. The additional cost of providing an additional volume of procedures or services. The additional cost may include additional fixed overhead costs as well as additional variable costs.

INDIRECT COST. Support services, such as hospital administration, medical staff office and public relations, which are not directly traceable to a particular service or procedure nor expensed in the producing department, but are expenses that apply to more than one direct service department.

INTERMEDIATE PRODUCT. One of several products (for example, inpatient nursing services) that is required to produce a final product (for example, normal delivery).

JOB COSTING. A methodology of costing applied in organizations where the resources consumed in producing individual products are easily traced.

JOINT COST. Costs associated with more than one product. Examples would include electricity or the depreciation of specific pathology equipment that can produce a variety of intermediate products.

LABOR STANDARDS. Expected amount of time for a typical employee to complete an assigned task. Sub-categories of standard labor measurements include applied hours, worked hours, paid hours, absent time, supervisory time and unmeasured time.

MARGINAL COST. The additional cost of one more unit, procedure or service. In concept similar to incremental cost, except incremental cost can refer to more than one additional unit of production.

NON-ASSIGNABLE COST. See ALLOCATED INDIRECT OVERHEAD or INDIRECT COST.

OPERATING COST. Direct material and direct labor costs.

OPPORTUNITY COST. The benefits relinquished when choosing an alternative use of resources.

OVERHEAD COST. See ALLOCATED INDIRECT OVERHEAD or INDIRECT COST.

PRIME COST. Total material and labor costs.

PROCESS COSTING. A methodology of costing used in organizations producing like products where, unlike job costing, it is not practical to track the resources consumed as each product is produced. Basically, an average costing process.

SEMI-FIXED COST. A cost that is fixed within a range of activity and which increases at workloads beyond that.

STANDARD COST. Normal predetermined unit cost computed on the basis of past performance, estimate or work measurement.

STATIC BUDGET. A budget projecting expenses at a single level of workload activity.

SUNK COSTS. Costs incurred in the past which are irreversible and not relevant to future decisions.

VARIABLE COST. A cost which varies in proportion to the level of activity.

80/20 RULE. A "rule of thumb" that 80 percent of resources are consumed in the process of producing 20 percent of the procedures or services.

Costing Methodologies: Job Costing vs. Process Costing vs. Relative Value Units

As in any other discipline, a theoretical understanding provides the foundation for actually constructing a cost accounting data base. The process of costing can be described as either job costing, process costing or a combination of the two.

In job costing, each job is the unit of activity to be costed. The activity is easily identified and costs are easily traceable. Examples of industries using job costing are accounting firms, ship builders, aircraft firms, job printing plants and architects. In each of these fields a job card or equivalent computer record can be used to document materials consumed and labor applied.

In contrast to job costing, process costing divides the costs for a stream of like products by the total units to determine, essentially, an average component cost per unit. Process costing is used in the chemical, food processing, paper, textile, and utility industries.

In the healthcare industry, time and materials are not tracked by the job. However, repetitive products are produced, such as PTCAs, gall bladder removals, etc. Yet the consistency of resources consumed for each like service (for example, PTCAs) can vary dramatically depending upon a variety of clinical considerations. Accordingly, the theory of job/process costing is selectively applied, depending upon the healthcare product being costed.

A third costing tool methodology, known as relative value units (RVUs) is already familiar to many clinical managers. The most recognized RVUs are CAP units used by pathology departments and designed by the College of American Pathologists.

RVUs are units of measure that recognize the relative differences in the consumption of resources between various procedures or services. For example, if a procedure A has a RVU value of 2 and a procedure B has a value of 4, it can be extrapolated that procedure B requires approximately twice the monetary resources as procedure A. These relative weights permit a costing process similar to process costing.

The RVU weights are determined by studies which are often conducted by industry groups. A major deficiency of industry-developed RVUs is that they are often based solely upon labor requirements and will not recognize the unique requirements of a particular hospital. However, they can serve as a basis of costing that still achieves higher quality results than a ratio of cost to charges.

More accurate RVUs are hospital-specific for both product and resources. For example, both a labor and material RVU may be developed for each cardio-diagnostic service. The more resource specific the RVU, the more accurate the costing.

Exhibit 4 illustrates in three steps how RVUs can be used for product cost allocation and estimation.

Cost Behavior Characteristics

Although the concepts of cost behavior may appear trivial, they are fundamental to cost accounting and are often misunderstood in practice.

To a significant extent, cost behavior is a function of time, resource management style, corporate goals and objectives as well as the organization's cost accounting objectives.

To determine standard and expected actual costs, one must know how costs react under various circumstances. There are two basic cost behavior patterns, fixed and variable. Fixed costs do not change as the level of measured activity or workload fluctuates (See Figure 3A). Variable costs will change in more or less direct proportion to the volume of activity (See Figure 3B).

It is perhaps easiest to understand these concepts by reviewing how they appear

Exhibit 4: RVU costing methodology for one department

Step 1

Procedure	RVU		Volume		Total RVUs
A	3	×	1000	=	3000
B	1	×	5000	=	5000
C	2	×	1000	=	2000
D	5	×	2000	=	10,000
				Total RVUs	20,000

Step 2

Total Dept. Direct Costs (#1)	Total Dept. Indirect Costs (#2)	Total Dept. RVUs (#3)	Direct Costs Per RVU (#1 ÷ #3)	Indirect Costs Per RVU (#2 ÷ #3)
$100,000	$50,000	20,000	$5.00	$2.50

Step 3

Procedure (#1)	RVU (#2)	Procedure Direct Cost (#2 × $5.00)	Procedure Indirect Cost (2 × $2.50)	Procedure Full Cost
A	3	$15.00	$ 7.50	$15.00 + $ 7.50 = $22.50
B	1	$ 5.00	$ 2.50	$ 5.00 + $ 2.50 = $ 7.50
C	2	$10.00	$ 5.00	$10.00 + $ 5.00 = $15.00
D	5	$25.00	$12.50	$25.00 + $12.50 = $37.50

graphically. Fixed costs have no relationship to volume. Depreciation is a good example of a fixed cost. Figure 3B demonstrates a pattern of variable costs. Notice that for variable costs, there is a direct relationship between volume and dollars spent. A good example of a variable cost is the relationship of contrast media expense to the volume of IVPs: when no IVPs are performed, the dollars spent on contrast media are zero.

A sub-category of variable costs is semi-fixed costs (Refer to figure 3C). Semi-fixed costs increase in steps as volume increases. Most technical and direct patient care labor costs behave as semi-fixed costs. For example, a 5 percent increase in workload may not necessitate a 5 percent increase in a department's staffing yet at a 10 percent workload increase, proportionate changes in staffing may be required. Over a year's time, it is reasonable to assume that semi-fixed costs will behave on average as variable costs; this is generally referred to as average variable costs.

One area of confusion in regard to cost behavior is committed and discretionary overhead expenses. For example, because of poor financial performance during a time of low sales (occupancy) a company may decrease discretionary fixed overhead expenditures, such as education and travel. One may conclude incor-

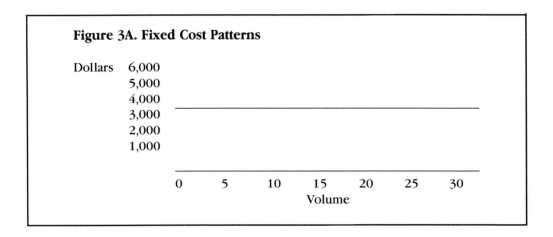

Figure 3A. Fixed Cost Patterns

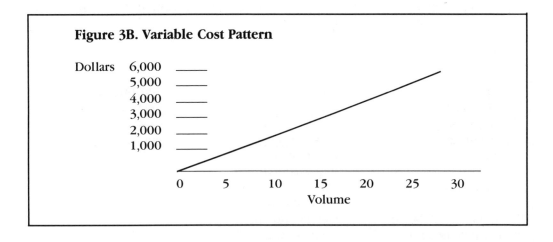

Figure 3B. Variable Cost Pattern

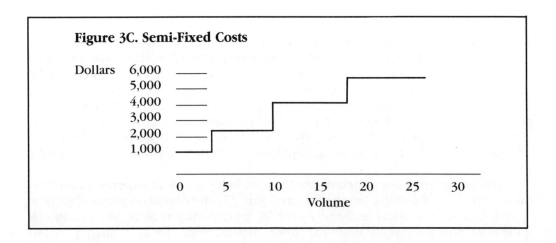

Figure 3C. Semi-Fixed Costs

rectly that the education expense is variable in relation to patient care workload because the amount of dollars was reduced during a time of lower volume. Actually, the fixed overhead expense was re-evaluated and a decision was simply made to reduce non-critical overhead expenses.

Quite often poor financial performance will result in the elimination of non-critical or perhaps even unnecessary discretionary fixed overhead expenses. Accordingly, overhead should never be regarded as a committed ongoing expense.

Many overhead expenses are even variable in the short term, with the incurred cost based upon some type of action, request or other type of transaction. However, there are committed expenses such as interest payments that cannot be eliminated except in the context of loan re-negotiation, repayment, bankruptcy, or company sale.

Thus, one sees that the classification of resources by cost behavior can be both confusing and transitory. In fact, the confusion arises from the transitory nature of cost behavior. The ideal cost accounting system should be able to respond to inquiries over both short-term and long-term planning horizons.

The following are examples of resources that are consumed according to the types of cost classifications discussed above.

Fixed	Variable	Semi-fixed
Management	Sutures	Technical labor
Supervision	X-Ray film	Patient care labor
Heating & light	Catheter tubes	Equipment repairs
Taxes	Patient food	
Dues/subscriptions	Registration forms	
Insurance on fixed assets	Malpractice insurance based upon usage	
Depreciation based upon useful life	Depreciation based upon usage	
Travel & auto expense	Consumables & other perishable items	

To reiterate, in practice it is important to recognize that the classification of expenses is dependent upon the cost accounting objectives. For example, the above classifications assume that: (1) all product lines are likely to be continued to be offered in the future and: (2) presumed volume changes are not likely to result in overhead structural changes. Within the hospital industry these assumptions are less reliable for long-term planning, as overhead requirements are subject to significant change, but they do serve as a basis for short-term planning, especially for addressing immediate cash flow and critical competitive concerns.

There are many ways to determine the cost behavior of an expense in relation to: (1) the unit of activity being measured and: (2) the cost accounting objective. These include statistical analysis, industrial engineering techniques, managerial judgment and interviews with executive management. From a quality, detail perspective, there is little doubt that industrial engineering will achieve the most accuracy.

However, in the healthcare industry there are advantages to combining the techniques of managerial judgment and quantitative studies. The main advantages are project efficiency and improved managerial skills in cost management and control. Because ancillary and patient care managers typically have been promoted from technician or patient care provider to supervisor to manager, they are usually extremely knowledgeable of the processes involved in providing their department's services. With the assistance of an experienced cost accountant or consultant, this knowledge can be applied to developing cost components. Any specific processes not known by the manager can be learned from supervisors and if necessary through time studies and other management engineering techniques.

In the short-term, such data should not produce materially different results than industrial engineering for such objectives as pricing decisions, program review, cost benefit analysis, utilization review by cost exception, PPO/HMO negotiations, flexible budgeting, etc. In fact, the increased managerial skills so developed may well be worth the modest loss of quality, not to mention the cost savings of not hiring a full-time industrial engineer.

However, an industrial engineer could make adjustments to the staff-estimated standards and provide suggestions on work simplification and productivity improvement. If an industrial engineer is already on staff, the organization will have an advantage in establishing standards to be used for cost accounting.

Chapter Four
Cost Accounting Process

The implementation of cost analysis within a department seems like a monumental task that can appear so overwhelming that few managers begin the process. However, if the process is broken up into smaller steps, it becomes easily achievable. Figure 4A conceptually diagrams the process of product service identification and costing.

Intermediate (Department) Product Costing

Steps 1 through 4 identify one of several common methods for associating department level costs with given intermediate products. All examples in the following steps will consist of three products: a chest X-ray (2 views), an upper GI and a gall bladder sonogram. At the conclusion of step 1 all services and products will be identified along with estimated or actual volumes, depending on whether standard or actual costing is being performed.

Step 1: Identify Product/Service. In a department, products and services will most often be identified by the already existing charge codes. For radiology this may include several hundred charge codes. Quite often there also will be patient and administrative services for which there are no charges or coding mechanisms. These non-charge items must be accounted for as well.

Step 2: Identify Variable Labor. To identify the labor costs for each product, it is necessary to examine the variable labor time associated with each identified product. Semi-fixed labor cost will be recognized as a variable cost based upon the assumption that volumes are likely to change sufficiently over the medium term (for example, during the course of a year) so as to proportionately influence the total cost of direct labor. The examples here (Figures 4B through 4I) include technical, clerical and transcription as variable labor.

Figure 4B outlines the estimated clerical, technical and transcription time for each of the three products under examination. Clerical time is assumed to be 10 minutes for each procedure. Technical time is assumed to be different for each procedure. Transcription time is again assumed to be the same for each procedure. In Figure 4B, one can see that the clerical time at $6.00 an hour translates to 10 cents per minute. This translation from hours to minutes is accomplished for both technical and transcription costs as well. The cost per minute is multiplied by the number of minutes for each procedure to give a total identified procedure cost for each component of the product.

When the initial labor time and cost estimates were made, they were an assessment of identified productive time. However, 100 percent of the employee's paid time is not spent in production. This non-productive cost of operating is

Figure 4A

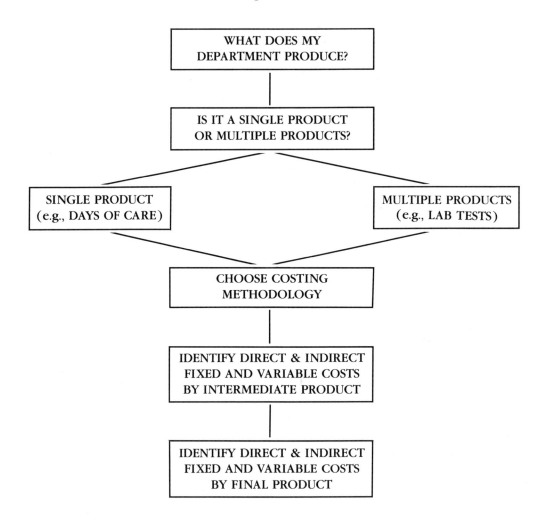

then allocated to each product. Figures 4C, 4D and 4E provide a method for including the direct non-productive dollars associated with each procedure. This allocation process recognizes the variability of non-productive expenses in relationship to changes in staffing requirements. An underlying assumption is that staffing requirements do change as a result of workload fluctuations.

In Figure 4C, we note that the total productive clerical cost is $38,000 based upon the identified time elements. This number is compared to the total variable labor costs in this area. In this example, we find that the total budgeted variable labor cost for clerical staff is $50,000 per year. This results in a $12,000 difference of non-productive time that was not accounted for in the direct time estimates. In order to be accurate in accounting for costs, the $12,000 must be allocated back to each procedure.

The $12,000 is divided by the $38,000 identified labor costs. This equates to a 32 percent ratio of non-productive to productive labor costs. Thus, each of the

Figure 4B. Traceable Productive Labor, Radiology Department

Procedures	Clerical	Technical	Transcriber
Chest X-ray (Two Views)	10 minutes × 0.10* = $1.00	8 minutes × 0.20† = $1.60	5 minutes × 0.15‡ = $0.75
Upper GI	10 minutes × 0.10 = $1.00	30 minutes × .20 = $6.00	5 minutes × 0.15 = $0.75
Ultrasound (Gallbladder)	10 minutes × 0.10 = $1.00	25 minutes × .20 = $5.00	5 minutes × 0.15 = $0.75
	* $6.00/hr. = $.10/min.	† $12.00/hr. = $.20/min.	‡ $9.00/hr. = $.15/min.

Figure 4C. Total Variable Clerical Labor, Productive & Nonproductive

Procedures	Volume	Total Clerical Identified	Total Variable Cost (per procedure)
Chest X-ray (Two Views)	20,000	$1.00 × 20,000 = $20,000	$1.00 × 1.32 = $1.32
Upper GI	10,000	$1.00 × 10,000 = $10,000	$1.00 × 1.32 = $1.32
Ultrasound	8,000	$1.00 × 8,000 = $ 8,000	$1.00 × 1.32 = $1.32
TOTAL	38,000	$38,000	

Total Actual Variable Clerical Salary Cost is equal to $50,000
Nonproductive = $50,000 minus $38,000 = $12,000

$12,000/$38,000 = 32% of productive labor costs unidentified.
Increase each productive cost by 32% to account for nonproductive costs.

identified labor costs must be increased by 32 percent to reflect the total standard variable cost.

Note that figures 4D and 4E perform the same computation for the technical and transcription staff. The methodology illustrated in figures 4C,4D and 4E is an example of developing hospital-specific labor RVUs based upon micro-costing studies.

After the variable labor component is identified for each employee classification, the individual components must be summed to assign a total variable labor component for each product line. This is illustrated in Figure 4F. The total labor cost per procedure is multiplied by the total volume of that procedure to result in the total cost required to produce that product. As a verification, this number is compared to the sum of the total budgeted salary costs.

Step 3: Identify Variable Materials Cost. The next task is to identify all variable material costs that are traceable to each individual product. The most significant costs in our example are film and contrast material. Figure 4G displays the traceable variable material costs for each of the identified product lines. Note that the same process was followed in identifying material costs as in identifying total variable labor costs.

The total identified cost per product is multiplied by the volume to indicate a total identified materials cost. The identified materials cost of $212,000 is com-

Figure 4D. Total Technical Variable Labor, Productive & Nonproductive

Procedures	Volume	Technical Identified	Total Variable Cost (per procedure)
Chest X-ray (Two Views)	20,000	$1.60 × 20,000 = $ 32,000	$1.60 × 1.70 = $ 2.72
Upper GI	10,000	$6.00 × 10,000 = $ 60,000	$6.00 × 1.70 = $10.20
Ultrasound (Gallbladder)	8,000	$5.00 × 8,000 = $ 40,000	$5.00 × 1.70 = $ 8.50
TOTAL	38,000	$132,000	

Total Actual Variable Tech Salary Cost equals $225,000

Nonproductive = $225,000 minus $132,000 = $93,000
$93,000/$132,000 = 70% productive labor costs unidentified.
Increase each productive cost by 70% to account for nonproductive costs.

Figure 4E. Total Transcription Variable Labor, Productive & Nonproductive

Procedures	Volume	Total Identified	Total Variable Costs (per procedure)
Chest X-ray (Two Views)	20,000	$.75 × 20,000 = $15,000	$0.75 × 1.40 = $1.05
Upper GI	10,000	$.75 × 10,000 = $ 7,500	$0.75 × 1.40 = $1.05
Ultrasound (Gallbladder)	8,000	$.75 × 8,000 = $ 6,000	$0.75 × 1.40 = $1.05
TOTAL	38,000	$28,500	

Total Actual Variable Transcription Salary Cost is equal to $40,000.
Nonproductive = $40,000 minus $28,500 = $11,500
$11,500/$28,500 = 40% productive labor costs unidentified.
Increase each productive cost by 40% to account for nonproductive costs.

Figure 4F. Variable Labor Summary

Procedure	Volume	Total Clerical/Technical/Transcription	Total
Chest X-ray (Two Views)	20,000	$1.32 + $ 2.72 + $1.05 = $ 5.09	$101,800
Upper GI	10,000	$1.32 + $10.20 + $1.05 = $12.57	125,700
Ultrasound (Gallbladder)	8,000	$1.32 + $ 8.50 + $1.05 = $10.87	86,960
	38,000		$314,460

Actual Total Salary Cost = $50,000 + $225,000 + $40,000 = $315,000
Difference between Actual of $315,000 and $314,460 is attributable to rounding.

Figure 4G. Traceable Variable Material

Procedures	Film	Contrast Media	Total Identified Cost Per Product	Volume	Total Identified Materials	Total Variable Cost (per procedure)
Chest X-ray (Two Views)	$ 4.00	$0.00	$ 4.00	20,000	$ 80,000	$ 4.00 × 1.05 = $ 4.20
Upper GI	$10.00	$2.00	$12.00	10,000	120,000	12.00 × 1.05 = $12.60
Ultrasound (Gallbladder)	$ 1.50	$0.00	$ 1.50	8,000	12,000	$ 1.50 × 1.05 = $ 1.58
Total				38,000	$212,000	

Total Actual Variable Materials Cost is equal to $222,600.
The difference of 5 percent between $222,600 and the $212,000 is attributable to such factors as waste, shrinkage and test repeats.
The total identified cost per product is increased by 5 percent.

pared to the actual materials cost of $222,600. The variance between the two is determined to be 5 percent. This 5 percent is allocated back to each individual product and leads to a total variable materials cost as indicated in the table.

Step 4: Identify Fixed Costs. Next the fixed costs must be allocated to each product. Fixed costs do not vary with volume. In a revenue department fixed costs typically are management and supervision salaries. The fixed cost must be totalled and then allocated to each product. In our example, the fixed costs were determined to be $50,000. The ratio of fixed costs to total variable costs is approximately 9 percent. This is determined by dividing the $50,000 fixed cost by the sum of the variable labor and materials costs.

Figure 4H illustrates how the fixed overhead is allocated. The total variable cost for each product is increased by the 9 percent fixed overhead allocation. This allocation process assumes that fixed costs exist to manage/support the direct production process in relation to the variable costs consumed.

Figure 4I summarizes the prior cost finding worksheets. It breaks down the cost of providing each service into its basic components of total direct variable and total direct fixed costs (excluding indirect allocations from overhead support departments).

Overhead Allocation

The preceding section described an allocation process for assigning departmental fixed expenses, such as the manager's salary, to a department's intermediate products. Other costs outside of the department must also be accounted for in determining an intermediate product's total fixed and variable cost. These expenses would include admitting, interest payments, administration, etc.

Most healthcare managers and Medicare reimbursement experts are familiar with the concept of assigning overhead expenses to revenue-producing departments. In procedural cost accounting it is necessary to assign those costs down to the intermediate product level.

Figure 4H. Fixed Overhead Allocation

Procedure	Volume	Total Variable Cost	Allocation of Fixed Overhead	Verification
Chest X-ray (Two Views)	20,000	$ 9.29	$ 9.29 × 1.09 = $10.13	$202,600
Upper GI	10,000	$25.17	$25.17 × 1.09 = $27.43	274,300
Ultrasound (Gallbladder)	8,000	$12.45	$12.45 × 1.09 = $13.57	108,560
			TOTAL	$585,460

$50,000/($222,600 + $315,000) = 9%
9% equal allocation of fixed overhead.

Actual = $222,600 + $315,000 + $50,000 = $587,600
The difference between $585,460 and $587,600 is
mostly attributable to rounding.

Figure 4I. Cost Summary

Procedure	Variable Labor	Variable Materials	Total Variable	Fixed Overhead	Total Full Cost
Chest X-ray (Two Views)	$ 5.09	$ 4.20	$ 9.29	$ .84	$10.13
Upper GI	$12.57	$12.60	$25.17	$2.26	$27.43
Ultrasound	$10.87	$ 1.58	$12.45	$1.12	$13.57

It should not be assumed that all overhead costs are fixed. For example, if certain full-time equivalents are assumed to be variable, subject to hiring and terminations based upon workload changes, then personnel costs that vary with the number of employees should be classified as variable. These personnel costs, such as Social Security contributions, may be expensed within the personnel department rather than in the employing department. Once identified, these variable overhead costs must be assigned at the procedure level.

However, caution must be used as some overhead costs can be either fixed or variable based upon management's cost philosophy. For example, if equipment is replaced based upon wear-and-tear criteria, the depreciation should be classified as variable, recognizing that each time the equipment is used a marginal amount of deterioration is taking effect. However, if the same equipment is replaced based upon technological obsolesence, depreciation is fixed because replacement is not based upon volume. Remember that fixed and variable cost characteristics are defined based upon cause (transactions) and effect (costs).

In allocating overhead expenses to the intermediate products it is suggested that each overhead department be separated into either two or four sub-departments. If two divisions are chosen, one would possess the department's fixed expenses and the other the variable expenses of the department. A four-way division would further separate the fixed and variable costs by labor and material. For example, outpatient registration would perhaps include the supervisor in the fixed labor registration account and the clerks in the variable labor account. Each of these overhead accounts would then be allocated to the relevant departments based upon statistics that reasonably measure a department's usage of those services. A second allocation would be necessary to allocate those costs down to the procedures/services themselves.

If an integrated cost accounting system is not in use, it would not be unreasonable to use the Medicare cost report step-down as a means for allocating costs down to the revenue-producing departments. A personal computer spreadsheet could then be used to allocate the department's indirect costs to the procedures based upon a direct allocation. Whereas indirect expenses may be allocated to the the receiving department based upon square footage, the indirect costs may be assigned to the department's products/services based on some other measure such as hours.

While other industries are very experienced in direct costing at the intermediate product level, the healthcare industry has extensive experience with indirect costing as a result of the requirements of the Medicare program's cost report. For this reason, this section has been relatively brief. The individual responsible for completing the organization's cost report can greatly contribute to this aspect of the cost accounting process.

After the allocation process, costing is complete at the department procedural level. At this time the following cost matrix should be available for any given intermediate product/service:

	Fixed	Variable	Total
Labor	x	y	x + y
Material	a	b	a + b
Total	x + a	y + b	x + y + a + b

Final Product Costing

Costing at the procedure level is primarily a labor-intensive effort using managerial judgment and micro-costing studies, but final product costing (for example, by DRG) is information system intensive requiring specific final product definitions.

Final product costing requires the development of a profile of intermediate products by the desired final product. The profile may provide the expected number of chest X-rays per admission and the average length of stay by clinical service as well as all the other procedures utilized by the patient. This profile can only be accessed by a case-mix computer system integrating the hospital's financial and medical records data base. The utilization of a case-mix system is described in Chapter 6.

Yet the most difficult conceptual part of final product costing is determining the product itself. The defined product is a function of the question being asked or the analysis being performed. For example, in the context of

Figure 4J. Final Product Costing by DRG #373: Normal Delivery Without Complications

Service Description	Average Utilization	Average Charges	Variable Cost Per Unit	Fixed Cost Per Unit	Variable Cost Per Case	Fixed Cost Per Case	Total Cost Per Case
Obstetrics–Nursing	2.5	$ 813	$125	$200	$313	$500	$ 813
Labor & Delivery	1.0	300	100	235	100	235	335
Fetal Monitoring	0.9	54	20	15	18	14	32
O/B Central Supply Kit	0.2	8	25	10	5	2	7
Miscellaneous	1.0	75	15	35	15	35	50
TOTAL		$1,250	$285	—	—	$786	$1,237

PPO contract negotiations, a med-surg day and the associated ancillary services may be the relevant final product if that is the unit of service purchased by the PPO.

The more difficult product definitions are in the realm of clinical utilization management. Currently, it is best initially to use DRGs as a defined final product. However, many physicians have correctly objected that the DRG assignments do not appropriately classify similar patients.

Although Medicare has not greatly refined its reimbursement system, other classification systems have been developed using severity of illness as a criterion for improved categorization. Several case-mix, cost accounting and decision support systems include alternative patient care classifications as part of the system capabilities. It is highly suggested that there be physician input into the choice of these alternative systems if the objective is physician review by profit/loss determination.

The costing of a final product, such as a normal delivery, is determined by multiplying the cost components for each of the intermediate products consumed in the process of delivering a final product by the total units utilized. For example, if a final product uses an average of 2.0 chest X-rays and the full cost of the exam is $25, the total cost of the associated exams is $50. This process is repeated for each intermediate product, which are finally summed to produce the total cost of the final product. The summation can be split into sub-totals so the total final product variable cost can be distinguished from the total full cost.

Figure 4J illustrates the cost finding for a final product, defined in this case as a normal delivery without complications.

Some Notes on Cost Finding

The objective of this chapter has been to present a methodology for cost finding at the intermediate and final product level. Now we will highlight five non-technical considerations to successful cost accounting.

1. Cost finding is unique in a hospital because each department is like a business unto itself, producing its own array of products. Conceptually, the cost accountant

is responsible for the costing of 30 to 50 different enterprises within one "hospital" or "healthcare provider." For a large medical center, the total potential products can easily exceed 8,000 items in a charge description master.

Accordingly, the cost accountant must recognize that each of the unique "manufacturers" (departments) within the hospital may require a different approach to costing. The accountant with limited costing experience should educate himself or herself about the production processes for each department before applying costing techniques.

2. If the hospital chooses to utilize existing finance or accounting staff for the costing endeavor, those individuals chosen should thoroughly read both academic and healthcare industry literature on cost accounting prior to beginning actual cost finding tasks (Refer to bibliography). The staff should also attend cost accounting seminars and develop contacts at other healthcare providers so they can learn from others' successes and mistakes.

3. Many hospitals have developed nursing patient classification systems as a tool for nurse staffing and budgeting. These classification systems recognize that within a patient unit different patients require various levels of nursing hours of care.

These classification systems are equally useful for intermediate product (nursing) costing and ideal for final product costing such as for DRGs. If possible these classifications should become part of a hospital's charge description master so that a cost accounting and a case-mix management system can utilize the additional data elements.

4. There certainly are arguments for initially utilizing spreadsheet software for cost finding during the first year of the process. However, for ongoing success, sophisticated cost accounting software on a powerful micro-computer, minicomputer or mainframe is required. A PC spreadsheet is slow, subject to error on memory requirements exceeding 640K, limited to cost finding and inadequate for discrete overhead allocations. A reputable cost accounting software module overcomes each of these limitations and provides cost accounting capabilities exceeding cost finding, such as variance analysis and integration capabilities into budgeting, case-mix management, and financial modeling systems.

5. If cost accounting is to be taken to its highest potential in a hospital setting, the acquisition of a comprehensive case-mix or decision support system should be seriously considered. Only with such a system is it possible to determine the cost of a final product such as a normal delivery or open heart surgery. The applications within such a system include budgeting "from the top down," financial modeling, accurate PPO-HMO profitability analysis, and physician bottom-line contribution determination, among others.

Chapter Five

Costing Information Systems

"Data is analogous to raw material, whereas information is data organized to be timely, relevant and meaningful."

It is not unusual for a hospital to have invested several millions of dollars of capital and labor into various information systems. Yet many of these systems fail to deliver basic information required for effective decision making.

This failure is attributable to systems primarily designed on a transaction basis for specific tasks such as billing, payroll and inventory tracking. Ironically, these same systems retain nearly all of the raw data required for improved decision making. The problem is the lack of integration among the various system components.

Until the time that these systems independently "talk" to each other, third-party systems are necessary to integrate the data into more meaningful information. These third-party systems minimally include case-mix (clinical) reporting and a cost accounting data base. Related capabilities include forecasting, modeling, PPO/HMO contract management and budgeting. Considering the millions of dollars invested in the existing systems, the additional cost of between $200,000 and $750,000 to be fully able to translate the data into timely, relevant and meaningful information is well worth the investment.

The objectives of this chapter are to: (1) explain the operations of a case-mix (clinical) reporting system, the most basic component of a decision support system, and (2) provide suggestions for the acquisition of a related system to develop a cost accounting data base.

There are several ways that these two systems, case-mix and cost accounting, can be grouped. One group is those that exist as a stand-alone, unattached system. These systems are self contained and do not interface with other systems. They have no compatability problems and no integration potential either. Often, a requirement for data duplication will exist for a user of this type of system. They use data that very likely already exists within another system. If you are at a facility where your existing systems give you nightmares, maybe stand-alone cost accounting and non-cost accounting systems would permit you to automate these additional functions without having to deal with the nightmares.

An integrated system should have the ability to interface with various systems, with the objective of either receiving or transmitting data, even if it is initially desired not to have comprehensive system integration. Figure 5A illustrates how data flows from the various related systems.

Figure 5A

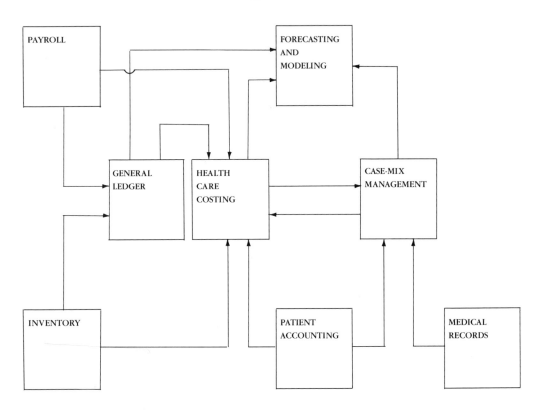

Case-Mix Management Systems

The hospital that does not have the use of a case-mix information system may be seriously handicapped in this very competitive healthcare market.

Today's marketplace demands much more sophisticated clinical and financial data than our industry has been accustomed to. Hospitals must now also be able to determine cost, profitability and resource utilization by defined products and specific patient characteristics. Such information provides the basis for effective PPO/HMO contracting, program planning, financial analysis and patient care medical management.

A case-mix computer system integrates information from the medical record, billing and cost accounting systems into a single data base. For each patient, the following key elements are tracked: procedures utilized, diagnoses, insurers, attending and admitting physicians and cost, charges, net revenue, contribution margin and net income amounts by defined level of intermediate and final product. Some systems will permit as many as 100 different elements to be tracked by each patient and to be summarized in many standard and ad hoc reports. Figure 5B lists some of these basic elements.

The development of a single integrated data base allows management to receive reliable answers to questions that previously could not be answered. Two examples of reports are profitability for each DRG for any particular physician and volume of patients by ZIP code by clinical service provided.

Figure 5B

Typical elements that can be tracked by case mix systems include:

Admission Date	Patient Identification
Age	Payer Type Classification
Birth Date	Payer Type by Specific Insurer
Cost & Charges	Peer Review Organization
Diagnosis—Admitting	Physician—Admitting
Diagnosis—Primary	Physician—Attending
Diagnosis—Secondary	Procedure Identification
Discharge Date	Sex
DRG	Source of Admission
Employer	Surgeon
Length of Stay	Surgical Procedure—Primary
Net Revenue	Surgical Procedure—Other
Occupation	ZIP Code

The success of a case-mix information system depends equally on the comprehensive and appropriate utilization of the system, the quality of the cost accounting data base and the case-mix software capability. Executive management must be aware of the system's capabilities and expected implementation schedules for achieving those capabilities. Critical is participation from the utilization review, financial management and the planning department personnel.

Utilization review can use the system for thoroughly reviewing physician practice patterns by comparing the specific hospital services requested by certain physicians for their patients within a given clinical product line with those requested by other physicians within the hospital. The financial management staff will be able to determine product line profitability and contract pricing criteria, among other applications. Marketing and planning staff will use both the demographic and financial data for developing short-term and long-term strategic plans. Since most of these applications are primarily of a financial nature, it is important that the cost accounting data included in the system be of high quality, thus increasing the credibility of the information provided to physicians and management.

In reviewing case-mix systems for acquisition, the hospital should consider user friendliness, quantity of standard reports, flexibility of ad hoc reporting, and ease of integration with the medical records, accounts receivables and intermediate product cost accounting systems, as well as limitations of number of patient elements to be tracked. Many vendors are offering case-mix, cost accounting, and other decision support modules which make data integration easier. Some mainframe vendors that sell general ledger and accounts receivables systems are also offering integrated cost accounting and case-mix clinical systems.

Cost Accounting System Selection Criteria

The purpose of this section is to list major considerations toward the purchase of a basic cost accounting system. By reviewing the following items and other readings in this book as well as discussions with vendors and other providers you should be well equipped to choose and implement a cost accounting system.

Specific Cost Accounting Considerations

1. Direct cost finding methodologies available (for example, Relative Value Units).
2. Indirect allocation methodologies available (for example, direct vs. step-down).
3. Ability to separate assigned overhead costs into fixed and variable cost components.
4. Ability to develop both standard and actual costs.
5. Standard cost variance analysis capabilities.
6. Quantity of service items that can be received from accounts receivable system.
7. Ability to add service items not included on accounts receivables system.
8. Classification requirements of cost centers into desired categories of direct patient care, support, overhead, etc.
9. Cost behavior categories available (for example, direct, indirect, fixed, variable, semi-fixed, labor, materials).

General System Reporting Considerations

1. Quantity and variety of standard reports.
2. Ad hoc reporting capabilities.
3. Visual layout of reports (including suitability for presentations).

Other Systems and Vendor Factors to Consider

1. Compatability with current hardware and software.
2. Description of system security.
3. User friendly, ease of use.
4. Availability of "help" screens.
5. Proposed system back-up methodology.
6. Error correction procedures.
7. Quality, completeness, and understandability of system documentation.
8. Initial price and on-going cost.
9. Vendor system maintenance and expected enhancements.
10. Length of start-up time.
11. Ability to transfer data to popular micro-computer spreadsheet applications software.
12. Language of software (for example, Basic).
13. Availability of source code for facility modification.
14. Number of product releases issued in the last two years.
15. Number of releases as a result of "bugs" and enhancements, as well as the nature of both the "bugs" and enhancements that necessitated additional releases.

16. Additional applications and modifications planned for the next three years.

17. Explanation of typical installation approach.

18. Availability of a "user group."

19. Number of products sold for each year since initial release.

20. Vendor background, including financial viability, diversity of products offered, research and development budget, support locations, and references.

Cost Accounting System Selection Summary

Since healthcare cost accounting and case-mix reporting is a new niche for computer vendors, caution needs to be exercised in choosing a system. It is best to become completely familiar with cost accounting before choosing a system. Developing cost accounting and case-mix reporting around a system's capabilities rather than choosing a system that best meets the hospital's immediate and future requirements will result in disappointment.

When beginning the vendor selection process, first specify your case-mix management and cost accounting system requirements and existing hardware and software. Translate this information into a Request for Proposal (RFP) to be sent to a list of potential vendors. Evaluate the responses to the RFP and carefully "interrogate" each vendor as to each special system's capabilities. Follow up by calling the vendors' prior installations (references) about general satisfaction and accuracy of responses to the RFP.

The group of individuals responsible for evaluating the various cost accounting software packages should include representatives from finance and information systems. The same group would evaluate the case-mix management systems but perhaps also include representatives from utilization review and marketing.

After reviewing each software package, the individual members of the evaluation group should complete worksheets rating individual software characteristics. Each rated item, derived from the RFP, would be weighted based upon the importance of the specific criteria being evaluated. The group chairperson would then total the results and internally develop a recommendation based upon objective (for example, rating worksheets) and subjective criteria.

The recommendation to management for the purchase decision should include a discussion of:

1. The original mission of the group (for example, evaluate cost accounting and case-mix management software).

2. The top three systems and their relative merits, including cost, benefits, description of the vendor, and key factors for their being the chosen system.

3. Brief description of rejected systems and why they were rejected. Should include comparative group scoring by system as compared to chosen system.

In summary, be knowledgeable about cost accounting before choosing a system and be certain that the system can deliver the applications required for improved decision making. Inquire about the vendors' long-term commitment to their products as measured by research and development expenditures. And do not be afraid to test the vendors' own knowledge about cost accounting and related applications.

Chapter Six

Cost Accounting Applications

Cost accounting is a commitment of time, energy, and resources. The endeavor should not merely be for the objective of reporting numbers but rather for increased control and improved profitability. This chapter highlights a few of the many applications of a quality cost data base.

Due to the complexity of each application, the discussion is expanded beyond cost accounting. This "holistic" approach recognizes that cost data is critical, but is certainly not the only information input required.

Factors Of Profitability

Although this section is brief, the business basics it discusses are as relevant to a small business as to a major corporation. An income statement format is used to communicate these basics. This approach will exemplify the role of cost accounting in achieving continued profitability.

The factors of profitability are few. Ironically, until now not many healthcare providers have actually attempted to quantify them.

These profitability factors can be conceptualized by breaking down the income statement into the equation:

$$\sum_{0}^{y} [(X)*(NR - VC)] - FC = PROFIT \ (LOSS)$$

Where: Y = the total types of product offered for sale
  X = the total volume of each product sold
  NR = the net revenue associated with each unique final product
  VC = the variable cost associated with each unique final product
  FC = the fixed costs associated with general operations that do not vary within expected workload changes.

The cost components identified as Y,X,NR,VC, and FC can be translated into the following operational policies for improved profitability.

$$\sum_{0}^{y} [(X)^{*}(NR - VC)] - FC = PROFIT \ (LOSS)$$

1. Increase the volume of products where the additional net revenue exceeds the variable (incremental) cost. Volume can be increased through PPO-HMO contracting, physician recruitment and other marketing strategies. A case mix system integrated with a cost accounting data base will provide the ability to identify the profitable product lines.

2. At all times achieve the highest price the marketplace will permit within the constraints of the strategic and marketing objectives of the organizaiton.

3. Increase productivity. Both cost accounting and productivity systems share similar labor data bases (for example, wage rates and standard times to complete tasks) creating efficiencies in simultaneous development of these systems. A productivity system can identify labor inefficiencies and be used as a tool for motivating increased productivity.

4. Reduce utilization of non-reimbursed services for the fixed price payers. A case mix system can be used for identifying inappropriate utilization of services by product line and physician.

5. Minimize the overhead requirements of the organization. Cost accounting can clearly identify the various cost components of an organization, facilitating reorganization and zero-based budgeting approaches to management.

Implementing these factors of profitability requires decisiveness and quality information. Cost accounting, case-mix and decision support systems can provide that data. An experienced cost accounting staff (or consultants) will ensure that those decisions are supported by quality information.

Cost Benefit Analysis

The loss of cost reimbursement and the erosion of charge-based payers have increased the financial risks associated with each new program and business opportunity. More than ever, executive management must be fully aware of the consequences of each major business decision.

Each new program should require a thorough cost benefit analysis to ensure that all quantitative and qualitative issues have been thought through, so as to result in the most intelligent decision.

Although financial cost is only one of several variables in completing a cost benefit analysis, it is certainly a major determinant of profitability. Cost accounting will increase the reliability of many analyses of profitability, particularly those concerned with either an expansion or a divestiture of existing services.

A complete cost benefit analysis will provide executive management with the following information:

Qualitative	Quantitative
Marketing Objectives	Net Income
Nursing Impact	Cash Flow
Ancillary Impact	Net Present Value
Support Services Impact	Return on Investment
Community Service	Sensitivity Analysis
Organizational Concerns	Debt Capacity Impact

Each of these issues should be addressed on a multi-year basis to identify both the changes internally and the continuing effect upon the competitive position of the institution. The desired thoroughness of the analysis will usually be a function of the resources and risk associated with the project.

Examples of programs requiring cost benefit analysis include fixed wing air ambulance transport, chemical dependency, mental health, nuclear magnetic resonator, organ transplants and any other services (with or without capital requirements) that generate revenue. Major expansion of existing programs should be viewed with the same level of critical review as new programs. Non-revenue producing investments such as plant replacement will be viewed more from the perspective of alternative decisions and the consequences of no decision.

Proposed programs that affect many departments are the most difficult to analyze. This is because many healthcare providers have not conducted pro-cedural-level cost accounting nor integrated the data into a case-mix management system. An integrated information base as described permits a high level of confidence in the cost and revenue results of the analysis. A quality case-mix system will also serve the marketing component of the review by providing demographic information on similar populations that currently utilize the hospital's services.

Although a cost benefit analysis will address all of the major issues, the most discussed and usually most critical section is the financial results. The financial review must not only show the direct impact on affected departments but also on the entire organization. The financial data will provide the change to the provider's income statement (net revenues over expenses) and overall cash flow. If a project requires significant start-up capital resources, it is quite possible for the two financial figures to differ significantly because of the treatment of depreciation or similar type expenses.

In today's environment of decreasing net revenue from the traditional sources of cash income, it is imperative that more emphasis be placed upon analysis that indicates changes in a provider's cash flow.

Since programs will continue to provide services for many years, any pro forma should account for several years of financial impact. Due to unknowns in the future, sensitivity analysis should be performed adjusting variables such as volume projections, payer type distributions and employee staffing. The additional effort to perform sensitivity analysis is typically minimal with the assistance of a personal computer and spreadsheet software such as Lotus 1-2-3.

To help the organization ration dollars among a variety of potential programs, it is useful to use objective financial criteria such as internal rate of return on investment and net present value. The net present value method discounts future net cash flows into a lump sum of current dollars so as to easily compare projects that have differing service lives, varying start-up requirements and annual returns. The discount (or interest) rate that is applied against the future cash flows is typically based upon the cost of capital and an organizationally desired rate of return adjusted to the perceived risk of the specific project.

Within the parameters of the cash flow assumptions, a net present value less than zero indicates that the investment will have a percentage return less than the chosen discount rate. The discount rate that results in a zero net present value is known as the internal rate of return.

The internal rate of return is similar to any other quoted return on an investment. For example, if a new program has a rate of return less than the money markets or treasury bonds, the appropriateness of the new program should be questioned and a lower risk alternative investment should be considered. Exhibit 5 presents most of the information that would be derived from a cost/benefit financial analysis.

Once the potential positive or negative financial returns of a program are known, it is appropriate to balance those returns against the marketing and operational issues. Quite often in today's intense competition for increased market share, financially marginal projects will be approved in order to achieve long-term strategic goals. However, under such a situation it is better to be aware of both the short-term and long-term financial consequences rather than base the decision solely on intuition and limited information.

Exhibit 5: Typical cost benefit analysis for program planning

	START-UP	YEAR 1	YEAR 2	YEAR 3–10
REVENUE				
Inpatient Revenue		300,000	450,000	600,000
Outpatient Revenue		100,000	150,000	300,000
Total Gross Revenue		400,000	600,000	900,000
Deductions From Revenue		100,000	180,000	360,000
NET REVENUE		300,000	420,000	540,000
EXPENSES				
Salaries & Wages		150,000	200,000	225,000
Benefits		37,500	50,000	56,250
Marketing		10,000	10,000	10,000
Other Non-Wage Expense		75,000	112,500	168,750
Equipment Depreciation		50,000	50,000	50,000
TOTAL EXPENSES		322,500	422,500	510,000
NET REVENUE OVER EXPENSES		(22,500)	(2,500)	30,000
Cash Flow Adjustments				
Minus Capital Acquisition Cost	(500,000)	—	—	—
Plus Capital Depreciation	—	50,000	50,000	50,000
NET CASH FLOW CHANGES	(500,000)	27,500	47,500	80,000
NET PRESENT VALUE:*	(62,107)			
INTERNAL RATE OF RETURN:	6.4%			

*Net present value is based upon a 9 percent discount rate. A negative net present value indicates that the program will generate an internal rate of return less than the criteria discount rate of 9 percent.

**A $500,000 investment producing the identical positive cash flows as the above example is equivalent to a 6.4 percent return.

Managed Care Contracting and Negotiations

Preferred provider organizations (PPOs) and health maintenance organizations (HMOs) are rapidly becoming a significant percentage of a hospital's clientele. At some institutions as much as 50 percent of the non-government gross revenue is represented by these alternative healthcare financing systems.

Effective PPO-HMO contracting requires staff that have the ability to communicate and negotiate effectively. That staff must also be supported by information systems providing cost, gross revenue, contracted discounts and profitability on existing contracts. This information is especially critical in renewal negotiations. Case-mix management and decision support systems can provide information on existing contracts as well as financial modeling capabilities for use in new contracts in the initial negotiation process.

There has been significant debate as to which cost is relevant for contract pricing: full (average) cost or incremental cost. For deciding upon the lowest acceptable price, there is little doubt that incremental cost determines the price floor. Both theoretical and practical experience reveal that the difference between a price above incremental cost and incremental cost itself provides a contribution toward fixed cost and net income. In other words, if a hospital loses patient business that provides a positive contribution margin (the difference between net revenue and incremental cost), the organization's net income and cash flow will likely decrease.

Incremental cost and pro forma profitability are much easier to determine for the per diem and per case arrangements that often characterize PPO contracts, than for HMO contracts that are often based upon a percentage of monthly subscriber capitation payments and risk pool distributions. HMO cost and profitability estimates simply are more volatile because the amount of future subscriber utilization is often unknown. Accordingly, pro forma HMO profitability analysis needs to be based upon actuarial studies and adjusted for a variety of potential utilization outcomes.

However, the practical usefulness of incremental cost is offset by the realistic objective to negotiate the highest price possible. In addition, approaching every contract and potential customer from a marginal or incremental basis carries the risk of severely underpricing services to the extent that the organization lacks the funds to pay the basic fixed costs of operations such as interest payments.

Market price is determined by the magnitude of the discount demanded by the PPO/HMO and the minimum price requirements of the healthcare providers.

Although market price is usually more relevant to negotiations than incremental cost, there can be times when cost is the critical factor. For example, in low occupancy markets the possibility of "net revenue" crashes exists. This can happen if hospitals collectively panic or collectively develop long-term strategic plans that are based upon short-term volume strategies, thus creating a ripe situation for a buyers' market for healthcare services. In such a situation each healthcare provider must know its incremental cost for that product line to be objectively aware of the lowest acceptable price and to be certain of the business and strategic value of maintaining or increasing patient market share.

Therefore, the value of entering a contractual relationship must be weighed against an organization's quantitative and qualitative opportunity costs as compared to the highest price one is able to negotiate in the marketplace. At this time, the organization's strategic objectives have a major impact upon the contracting decision process.

In all negotiating situations it is best to determine the highest price the PPO/HMO will accept before the PPO/HMO terminates discussions or opens talks with your competitor. Estimating the best market price is learned through experience. After 10 or more signed contracts and various negotiations, a reasonable knowledge of the highest price can be developed. However, this assumes that the hospital's contract negotiator is always achieving the best price possible. Only by knowing your competitor's prices can you be assured that you have achieved the best price.

Once the hospital has a reasonable grasp of cost and market price, it must use this information to fullest advantage. To begin, the hospital should never accept or propose a bid below incremental cost, unless there is an overriding strategic or marketing objective for which the institution is willing to accept a negative cash flow.

If the objective is to seek the highest price, it is best to propose bids no lower than market price. However, each hospital may have individual characteristics that can result in negotiated prices higher or lower than the average PPO/HMO prices for the community. Accordingly, the bid should reflect the hospital's unique niche in the local healthcare market and the perceived need of the PPO/HMO to include the hospital in its PPO/HMO network. Given the right set of circumstances, it is even possible in today's highly competitive marketplace to negotiate prices at a minimal discount from charges.

It is important that the bid structure reflect the variety of services offered by the institution. A single per diem may be appropriate for a low intensity community hospital. However, an all-inclusive per diem for a tertiary care center carries the risk of a higher than expected acuity by the PPO population. To minimize risk, a tertiary care center should consider proposing separate prices for trauma, burn, neonatal, ICU and cardiovascular services. Also, if an all-inclusive obstetric package is requested, the hospital may want to counter-offer with both a normal and a Caesarean price.

It needs to be mentioned that HMO contract negotiations differ most from PPO arrangements because subscriber capitation payments represent most of the hospital's HMO net revenue. Although some HMOs are reluctant to negotiate the percentage of the capitation to be provided to the hospital, opportunities for negotiation still exist. This includes a payment floor per enrollee to protect against the possibility of subscriber-price competition among the community's HMOs. Other negotiable items are HMO versus hospital versus physician patient service obligations as well as the risk pool formula itself. Another option is to negotiate a PPO-type per diem arrangement versus share of capitation. However, the per diem option does not align the hospital and IPA incentives with clinical utilization.

There may be opportunities for which a hospital will accept less than market price. Often a lower price is accepted in exchange for exclusivity for all or selected services. The exclusivity guarantees a volume base along with the certainty that the local competitor will lose market share. If exclusivity is a goal, the hospital should pursue a multi-year contract to lock out competitors.

Contract price negotiations are often difficult when the PPO/HMO refuses to accept rates that the healthcare provider believes are fair and reasonable to both parties. At that point the negotations almost become a poker game: it becomes important to determine whether the PPO/HMO negotiator is bluffing. Calling the negotiator's bluff has definite risks as does accepting the offered prices.

Cancelling negotiations until the PPO/HMO is willing to provide a better price is an acceptable strategy but should be used selectively. Before considering the strategies of stalling or cancelling negotiations, seriously consider the financial (for example, cash flow) and marketing consequences of losing the contract.

Contract negotiations should not center around price to the exclusion of the services being offered. Quite often unique services, community support and a high quality of care can generate a higher price. Sometimes the PPO/HMO will suggest a reasonable price in recognition of these considerations. However, the hospital should not be bashful nor assume a full awareness by the PPO/HMO negotiator. The hospital should highlight the unique and valued services it provides to the community. Most importantly, the hospital should attempt to develop an open and honest relationship with the PPO/HMO negotiator, who may well be sitting at the bargaining table many times more over the years.

Most of this section has discussed initial negotiations. In these "primary" negotiations the PPO/HMOs seem to have the advantage because it is known, but perhaps not said, that the patient business will go elsewhere if the contract is not signed by the hospital. However, in renewal negotiations (for example, after one year) the advantage shifts to the hospital because the PPO/HMO's subscribers have developed linkages to the hospital and its physicians. The PPO/HMO at that time does not desire to break that linkage and potentially lose subscribers. The quality of the network is part of the product being sold by the PPO/HMO to the consumer. Accordingly, the hospital can be much more aggressive in negotiating better payment after the first year, particularly if the initial rate was lower than market price.

Prior to and after signing contracts it is critical that several systems be in place, including cost accounting, decision support, case-mix management, and daily logging. A bare minimum system will include a logging software package typically managed by the business office. This system should be able to track volume and revenues from all prospective payment payers including Medicare, Medicaid, PPOs and HMOs. The available information will provide the basis for ensuring timely payment by the insurers as well as the ability to accurately determine the contractuals and net revenue on the financial statements.

A comprehensive HMO/PPO logging system will include the following report features:

- —Detailed recording of all pertinent contract factors
- —Determination of contractual allowances
- —Contract ad hoc reporting
- —Interface capability with accounts receivable system (typically UB-82)
- —Accounts receivable follow-up reports as well as A/R aging
- —Comparison of computed expected payment based upon contractual terms as compared to actual payment summarized on remittance advice
- —Breakdown of clinical classifications by payers as described by contract payment criteria (for example, Med-Surg, ICU, Cardiovascular)

A cost accounting system integrated with a case-mix management system provides an excellent tool for cost and profit (contribution margin) analysis by contract. In addition, a case-mix management system provides a wealth of information to the marketing, planning, finance and utilization review departments through the applications of a data base that contains clinical, financial and demographic information for each patient admission, visit and contract payment criteria. In most cases, the PPO or HMO has excellent data from which to negotiate. Accordingly, the hospital must be armed with equivalent data to understand the impact that each proposed price structure will have upon its profitability.

The people component of the systems is as important to the success of the contracting function as are the automated components. Typically, either the marketing or the finance department will be responsible for managing contracting activities. Quite often the responsibilities will be shared between the two departments.

How the function is structured depends upon the negotiation, sales, and analytical skills of the respective department members. A critical element to the structure determination is team player attitude. It is important that some individual coordinate the contracting process between admitting, utilization review, the physicians, billing and collections, and the PPO itself. In many institutions a finance or marketing staff member has been designated as a full-time contract manager or director to manage these daily responsibilities.

If the hospital contracts with HMOs on a "full risk" or capitated basis, systems must be in place to track the capitation's income, patient charges and purchased medical services to compute accurately the distribution of the risk pool surplus between the IPA and the hospital. In addition, it is critical to establish and maintain a close working relationship with the IPA medical groups so that the hospital has input into utilization review decisions. Currently, it is becoming common for administrative personnel to be responsible for both hospital contracting and IPA management.

Without these systems in place the contracting efforts may enter turbulent political waters. Board members, corporate staff and administrators will want to know the status of each contract. The PPOs will often incorrectly pay for a claim. Auditors will question the validity of the financial statement contractuals. If these embarrassing and costly situations are to be avoided, concurrent and historical systems and an appropriate organizational structure must be in place and operating.

The objective of this section has been to provide basic but not comprehensive guidelines for contracting. Effective contracting requires organizational communication, excellent interpersonal skills and common business sense. If all of this is combined with a strong sense of direction, as defined by a strategic plan, a hospital will have a competitive advantage over any hospital less equipped.

Cost Accounting and Flexible Expense Budgeting

Most budgets are based upon a given level of projected activity. Any significant variance from the budgeted volume projections limits the usefulness and credibility of the fixed budget. In addition, any positive reinforcement or negative response to actual results as compared to budget may be based upon faulty logic, if the results are not adjusted for workload variances.

A flexible budget recognizes that the primary objective of the department manager is to manage resources so as to provide some level of quality outcomes within a given level of activity (workload). The flexible budget adjusts those costs that vary with workload. For example, in an inpatient unit the standard cost of direct labor may be $150 per day and the fixed cost of management may be $3,000 per month. Assuming 300 patient days during the month, the expected labor expense would be $48,000 or ($150x300) + $3000.

Adjusting the budget to actual activity eliminates the question of how much of the budget variance is attributable to unexpected volume projections and concentrates on the expertise of managing costs in relation to customer demand. However, the cost of providing a more relevant budget is the development of the data base to retrospectively adjust the budget.

The sophistication of flexible budgets varies widely. Most organizations will vary costs by a broad measure of activity such as the volume of procedures for a given department. This is effective as long as the mix of procedures does not change.

Pathology departments will quite often use CAP (College of American Pathologist) units as a means for varying budgets. However, industry developed units quite often are based upon labor requirements only and do not reflect the unique characteristics of a specific institution.

The cost data developed at the procedure level will provide the most accurate flexible budget. The example on the next page illustrates the use of procedural cost accounting in a flexible budgeting application.

In the example, the relevant variable cost (for example, labor) associated with a unique product is multiplied by the respective volume to provide the total variable cost for that item. The process is repeated for each of the costed items, totaled, and added to the fixed cost of the department providing the total expected cost for the actual volume of workload experienced. Obviously, the process is quite simple for a department of few items. For a large department, a spreadsheet such as Lotus 1-2-3 will perform very effectively. However, if the finance/accounting department desires to centralize the process for all departments, much more sophisticated software will be required.

Cost Data

	Variable Labor Cost per Unit	Variable Material Cost per Unit
Procedure X	$ 2.00	$5.00
Procedure Y	$10.00	$1.00
Procedure Z	$ 5.00	$1.00

Fixed Management Salary Cost per Month: $3,000

Volumes

	CASE A	CASE B	CASE C
Procedure X	1,000	500	2,500
Procedure Y	2,000	2,000	500
Procedure Z	3,000	3,000	1,500

Flexible budgets

Salaries	$40,000	$39,000	$20,500
Materials	10,000	7,500	14,500
Total	$50,000	$46,500	$35,000

Variance Cost Analysis for Resource Management and Control

Standard costs are a management tool that can be used for controlling costs, measuring efficiencies, motivating cost reductions, assigning costs to inventory for financial reporting purposes, establishing budgets and forming the basis for bids and contracts.

This section concentrates on the application of standard costs for control objectives. In a business, there must be a means to explain the difference between actual costs and some predetermined standard. Without this variance explanation, a crucial management control and accountability tool is missing. Standard cost variance analysis not only provides a means to identify the cause of inefficiencies but also creates goals for middle management.

Four basic standard variance analysis techniques are discussed below: materials price variance, materials quantity variance, labor efficiency variance and labor rate variance.

Currently, the level of precision of variance analysis as applied in a hospital will not approach that of a manufacturer producing a single product. However, it is possible now to begin using similar variance analysis techniques as an additional tool for resource management and as a training basis in anticipation of improved software and more sophisticated product determination and analysis.

The following variance analysis examples provide a preview of the analytical techniques health care can expect in the near future.

Materials Price Variance. Material price standards are based upon the expected cost of materials for production during a given time period. Primarily, the responsibility for the acquisition cost of materials is given to the Materials Management department. Although material prices are determined by the marketplace, purchases can be made in large volume to achieve price savings, bid quotations can be obtained from several vendors, accounts payables can take advantage of early payment discounts, etc.

A price variance results if the price for goods differs from an expected standard. This variance is computed as follows: The $2,000 materials price variance is favorable because expected cost per unit is $.20 less than the expected purchase price of $2.50.

	Volume	×	Unit Cost	=	Variance
Actual quantity purchased	10,000	×	$2.30 actual	=	$23,000
Actual quantity purchased	10,000	×	$2.50 std.	=	$25,000
Total Materials Price Variance	10,000		$(.20)		$(2,000)

Materials Quantity Variance. Materials quantity variance is determined by comparing the cost of the actual usage of material in the production process with the expected cost of usage. The department manager who orders items from the materials management department is responsible for controlling waste, spoilage, theft and otherwise for efficient use of resources. The quantity variance is computed as follows:

	Volume	×	Unit Cost	=	Variance
Actual quantity purchased	10,000	×	$2.50 std.	=	$25,000
Standard quantity purchased	9,000	×	$2.50 std.	=	$22,500
Total Materials Quantity Variance	1,000		$2.50		$ 2,500

The unfavorable variance of $2,500 was caused by the purchase of 1,000 more units of materials than was expected.

Labor Efficiency Variance. The labor efficiency variance is determined by comparing the actual hours worked with the expected hours and determining the financial consequence based upon a standard labor wage rate. The variance is computed as follows:

	Volume	×	Unit Cost	=	Variance
Actual hours worked	1,000	×	$12.50 std.	=	$12,500
Standard hours allowed	900	×	$12.50 std.	=	$11,250
Total Labor Efficiency Variance	100		$12.50		$ 1,250

The unfavorable variance of $1,250 was caused by the usage of 100 hours more labor than expected.

Labor Rate Variance. The labor rate variance is similar to the materials price variance in that it is a measure of the management of a resource input (labor) on a per unit basis. The rate variance is measured as follows:

	Volume	×	Unit Cost	=	Variance
Actual hours worked	1,000	×	$11.00 actual	=	$11,000
Actual hours allowed	1,000	×	$12.50 std.	=	$12,500
Total Labor Rate Variance	1,000		($ 1.50)		($ 1,500)

The favorable result of $1,500 is easily associated with the $11.00 actual hourly rate versus an expected $12.50 per hour wage.

Bibliography

Arnstein, William E., *Direct Costing.* New York, New York: Amacom, 1980.

Burik, David, "Hospital Cost Accounting: Strategic Considerations," *Healthcare Financial Management,* February 1985, pp 19–28.

————, "Hospital Cost Accounting: A Basic System Approach," Ibid, March 1985, pp 58–64.

————, "Hospital Cost Accounting: Implementing the System Successfully," Ibid, April 1985, pp 76–88.

————, "Hospital Cost Accounting: Finding the Software Solution," Ibid, May 1985, pp 76–84.

Cleverley, William O., *Topics in Healthcare Financing Product Costing,* Frederick, Maryland: Aspen Systems Corporation, 1987.

Computers in Healthcare: 1986 Market Directory, Englewood, Colorado: Cardiff Publishing, 1986.

HFMA & Deloitte Haskin & Sells, *Cost Accounting: The State of the Art in Hospitals,* Oakbrook, Illinois: HFMA Professional Publications, 1986.

Deason, Green M., *Topics in Healthcare Financing: Flexible Budgeting,* Germantown, Maryland: Aspen Systems Corporation, 1979.

Herkimer, Allen G. Jr., *Topics in Healthcare Financing: Improving Productivity,* Germantown, Maryland: Aspen Systems Corporation, 1977.

Horngren, Charles T., *Introduction to Management Accounting,* Englewood Cliffs, New Jersey: Prentice-Hall, 1984.

Kukla, Steven F., *Cost Accounting and Financial Analysis for the Hospital Administrator,* Chicago, Illinois: American Hospital Publishing, 1986.

Mowen, Maryanne M., *Accounting for Costs as Fixed and Variable,* Montvale, New Jersey: National Association of Accountants, 1986.

Newton, Green W., *Internal Reporting & Analysis,* Marina Del Rey, California: Malibu Publishing, 1984.

Article Adaptations

Several chapters of this primer were adapted, modified and expanded upon from published articles written or co-authored by the author, Jeffrey A. Gottlieb. The author gratefully acknowledges the permission of the respective publishers for using the following articles as a contribution toward the development of this primer.

Chapter	Pages	Adapted Article
2	5–10	Gottlieb, Jeffrey A. and Matthew Stellato "Planning for Successful Implementation of a Cost Accounting System," Newsbrief, Southern California Chapter, HFMA December 1987/January 1988, pages 4, 10, 11
3 4	28–32 33–40	Gottlieb, Jeffrey A. and Suskin, Steven W. "Applications and Rewards of Cost Accounting: A Practical Approach," *Radiology Management*, Sudbury, Massachusetts: American Hospital Radiology Management. Summer/July 1986, pp 35–41
6	57–59	Gottlieb, Jeffrey A. "Incremental Cost and Profitability: Micro-Economics Revisited," *Hospital Cost Accounting Advisor*, Frederick, Maryland: Aspen Systems Corporation December 1986 Pages 1, 5–7
6	65–71	Gottlieb, Jeffrey A. "The Strategies and Negotiations Involved in PPO Contracting," *Healthcare Financial Management*, Oakbrook, Illinois: Healthcare Financial Management Association, May 1987, Pages 86–88.

Acknowledgements

The author wishes to thank the following individuals for their contributions to this publication:

Steve Brandman, Consultant
(Laventhol & Horwath, Los Angeles, California)

Judy Carney, Manager, Information Systems
(Presbyterian Intercommunity Hospital, Whittier, California)

Philip Gross, Consultant
(Laventhol & Horwath, Los Angeles, California)

Eytan Ribner, Partner
(Blumberg, Ribner & Company, Los Angeles, California)

Matthew Stellato, Regional Marketing Manager, Decision Support Services
(HBO & Associates, Los Angeles, California)

Paul Wales, Director—Managed Care Programs
(Presbyterian Intercommunity Hospital, Whittier, California)

In addition, the author wishes to extend his appreciation to those individuals who recognized the importance of cost accounting applications in the healthcare industry and contributed toward the management (cost) accounting experiences of the author. These individuals include:

Kent Badger, Chief Operating Officer
(Presbyterian Intercommunity Hospital, Whittier, California)

Robert Dickler, Chief Executive Officer
(University Hospital, Minneapolis, Minnesota)

Morris Freiling, Assistant Director, Ancillary Services
(University Hospital, Denver, Colorado)

Edward Sorenson, Chief Financial Officer
(San Bernardino Community Hospital, San Bernardino, California)

David Wood, Senior Associate Director and Chief Financial Officer
(University Hospital, Denver, Colorado)

About the Author

Jeffrey A. Gottlieb, M.S., is President of Gottlieb & Gottlieb, a healthcare financial management consulting firm specializing in program and capital planning, cost accounting, and HMO/PPO contract management review. Mr. Gottlieb was Director of both Finance Operations and Product Cost Accounting at a 358-bed regional medical center in Whittier, California. His other professional experience includes Manager of Financial and Cost Analysis at a 398-bed university teaching hospital in Denver, Colorado, and healthcare financial consultant at a major accounting firm in Los Angeles, California.

Mr. Gottlieb earned a Masters of Science degree in public policy and management from Carnegie-Mellon University's School of Urban and Public Affairs in Pittsburgh, Pennsylvania, and a Bachelor of Arts degree in political science from the University of California, San Diego. He has also completed coursework at the Carnegie-Mellon Graduate School of Industrial Administration, University of Pittsburgh School of Public Health and the University of Colorado, Denver School of Business Administration. Throughout his education, Mr. Gottlieb has focused on management (cost) accounting, finance, cost/benefit (investment) analysis, healthcare delivery and healthcare public policy.

Jeffrey A. Gottlieb has published several articles covering cost management, cost accounting and HMO/PPO contract management. He is a member of the National Association of Accountants and the Healthcare Financial Management Association as well as a faculty member of the University of La Verne Graduate School Health Care Management Program.